COOKBOOK FOR ILEOSTOMY

Ileostomy Meal Plan

Elevate Your Culinary Experience And Health Simultaneously With This Nutritious Meal Friendly Guide

DR. SOFIA SILAS

Table of Contents

CHAPTER ONE

Introduction

Living with an ileostomy may bring several obstacles, especially in terms of good nutrition and meal planning. An ileostomy is a surgical operation in which the small intestine is diverted via an abdominal orifice known as a stoma.

This change in the digestive tract may affect how the body absorbs nutrients from meals, thus people with ileostomies must be very mindful of their diet and eating habits. In this topic, we will look at ileostomy, the necessity of a healthy diet, necessary nutrients for ileostomy patients, meal planning, grocery shopping suggestions, and cooking methods designed specifically for people with ileostomies.

Understanding Ileostomy

An ileostomy is often used to treat inflammatory bowel disease, colorectal cancer, and other digestive problems. During this treatment, the surgeon makes a stoma by passing a section of the small intestine through the abdomen wall.

Waste from the small intestine is subsequently sent via the stoma to an external pouch, avoiding the colon and rectum. While an ileostomy may greatly enhance the quality of life for those with certain medical issues, it also necessitates lifestyle changes, notably in terms of food and nutrition.

Benefits Of A Healthy Diet

Maintaining a varied and healthy diet is critical for general health and well-being, particularly for those who have an ileostomy.

A diet high in important nutrients aids in healing, lowers the risk of problems and supports proper digestion. Furthermore, an appropriate diet may help control symptoms like diarrhea, dehydration, and electrolyte imbalances, all of which are typical concerns among ileostomy patients. Individuals who concentrate on nutrient-dense meals may improve their nutritional intake and quality of life after ileostomy surgery.

Essential Nutrients For Ileostomy Patients

Ileostomy patients may have special dietary requirements owing to changes in the structure and function of their digestive tract. Some vital nutrients that demand attention are:

1. Protein is essential for tissue regeneration and wound healing, especially for those recuperating from surgery. Lean meats, poultry, fish, eggs, dairy products, lentils, and tofu are excellent sources of protein.

2. Ileostomy patients may have dehydration and electrolyte abnormalities owing to increased fluid loss via the stoma. Staying hydrated requires consuming enough fluids, such as water, electrolyte-replenishing beverages, and clear broths.

3. Soluble fiber sources, such as oats, bananas, cooked vegetables, and peeled fruits, might help control bowel movements and avoid diarrhea in patients with an ileostomy. However, excessive insoluble fiber can induce blockages.

4. Adequate consumption of vitamins and minerals, including vitamin B12, calcium, iron, and potassium, is essential for good health and vitality.

Dietary supplements may be required to correct any deficiencies, particularly if specific nutrients are not effectively absorbed owing to the ileostomy.

Plan Meals For Ileostomy

Meal planning is essential for ensuring that people with ileostomies meet their nutritional requirements while eating a diverse and pleasant diet. Here are some suggestions for preparing ileostomy-friendly meals:

1. Eat smaller, more frequent meals to avoid intestinal overload and pouch leaks.

2. Choose readily digested meals, such as prepared fruits and vegetables, delicate meats, and

well-cooked grains, to reduce stoma discomfort.

3. Experiment with various cooking methods, such as pureeing, steaming, baking, and grilling, to improve food palatability and digestibility for those with ileostomy.

CHAPTER TWO
Grocery Shopping For Ileostomy-Friendly Ingredients

Navigating the grocery store aisles may be difficult, particularly when attempting to find items that are appropriate for an ileostomy diet. Here are some food-buying tips:

1. Read labels carefully. Pay close attention to the ingredients list and nutritional information on packaged goods to avoid anything that may aggravate digestive difficulties or pain.

2. Choose nutrient-dense staples such as whole grains, lean meats,

fresh fruits and vegetables (without rough skins or seeds), calcium and vitamin D-fortified dairy alternatives, and healthy fats like avocados and almonds.

3. Caution: Pre-packaged and convenience meals may include additives, preservatives, or extra salt, which may be troublesome for those with ileostomy. Choose less processed choices wherever feasible.

Cooking Tips For Ileostomy Meals

Adopting proper cooking procedures may significantly improve the digestibility and pleasure of meals for those who have an ileostomy. Here are some culinary ideas to consider:

1. Avoid fried and spicy meals, since they might be difficult to digest and cause stomach discomfort. Instead, use moderate cooking techniques such as baking, broiling, steaming, and poaching.

2. Peel and boil fruits and vegetables: Remove skins, seeds, and rough fibers to improve digestion and reduce stoma irritation. Cooking or pureeing food may also improve its digestion.

3. Consume probiotic-rich foods to maintain healthy gut flora and aid digestion. To promote digestive health, include fermented foods like yogurt, kefir, sauerkraut, and kimchi in your diet.

To maintain maximum health and well-being while living with an ileostomy, food, and nutrition must be carefully monitored.

Understanding the special nutritional demands of people with ileostomies and employing meal planning, grocery shopping, and cooking procedures may help you enjoy a diverse and enjoyable diet while avoiding digestive pain and difficulties.

Individuals who have had ileostomy surgery may flourish and retain a good quality of life with the correct direction and care.

Adapting Recipes For Ileostomy-Friendly Cooking

Living with an ileostomy, whether temporary or permanent, frequently requires dietary changes to guarantee comfort and health. An ileostomy is a surgical procedure that includes establishing a stoma in the abdomen through which waste exits the body and enters a pouch.

Certain foods might affect digestion and stool consistency, so it's critical to adjust recipes for ileostomy-friendly cooking. We'll look at breakfast choices, lunch alternatives, supper dishes, and snacks/appetizers designed specifically for people with ileostomy.

Breakfast Ideas For Ileostomy

Starting the day with a healthy and easy-to-digest breakfast is critical for those with ileostomies. Choosing low-fiber meals may reduce the likelihood of blockages and discomfort. Consider including the following breakfast options:

1. Smoothies: Combine ripe bananas, yogurt, almond milk, and berries for a tasty and digestible morning smoothie. Avoid adding fibrous fruits such as apples and oranges.

2. Scrambled eggs are a protein-rich food that can be easily digested. For added taste and nutrition, mix it with grated cheese or chopped spinach.

3. Oatmeal: Cooked oatmeal with water or lactose-free milk is a warm and satisfying breakfast

option. Instead of nuts or seeds, try honey, cinnamon, or mashed bananas.

4. Top plain, low-fat yogurt with soft fruits such as ripe peaches, mashed berries, or stewed apples to enhance taste and nutrients without adding too much fiber.

CHAPTER THREE

Lunch Options For Ileostomy

For lunch, choose light yet filling dishes that will not induce discomfort or extra gas. Here are some lunch alternatives appropriate for someone with an ileostomy:

1. To make a chicken or turkey sandwich, use soft white bread and thinly slice cooked chicken or turkey. If tolerated well, top with lettuce and a piece of cheese.

2. Make a homemade vegetable soup using well-cooked veggies such as carrots, zucchini, and potatoes. Avoid adding rough or

fibrous veggies, and try mixing the soup to aid digestion.

3. Tuna Salad: Combine canned tuna, mayonnaise, and finely chopped celery for a protein-packed salad. Serve it on a bed of lettuce or among soft crackers.

4. Rice Bowl: For a balanced and easy-to-digest lunch, top cooked white rice with lean protein like grilled fish or tofu, as well as steamed veggies like carrots and green beans.

Dinner Recipes For Ileostomy

Dinner provides a chance to eat tasty yet mild dishes that will not irritate digestive troubles. Here are some meal dishes appropriate for someone with an ileostomy:

1. Pair baked fish with creamy mashed potatoes for a nutritious and easy-to-digest meal. fish is rich in omega-3 fatty acids.

2. Top soft pasta shapes like penne or farfalle with a mild marinara sauce prepared from ripe tomatoes and herbs. Avoid using too much garlic or onion, since these might be difficult to stomach.

3. Roast Chicken with Steamed Vegetables: Serve tender chicken with steamed broccoli, cauliflower,

and carrots. Remove the skin to lower fat content, if required.

4. Quinoa Stir-Fry: Cook quinoa until fluffy and add soft veggies like bell peppers, mushrooms, and snap peas. Add cooked shrimp or tofu for protein and flavor.

Snacks And Appetizers For Ileostomy

Snacks and appetizers may be had in between meals to maintain energy levels while avoiding digestive problems. Here are some suggestions for ileostomy-friendly foods.

1. Spread smooth peanut butter over rice cakes for a low-fiber, easy-to-digest snack.

2. Cottage Cheese with Pineapple: Combine cottage cheese and canned pineapple pieces for a protein-packed snack with a touch of sweetness.

3. Hard-boiled eggs are a handy, protein-rich snack.

4. Rice Crackers with Hummus: Pair rice crackers with creamy hummus for a tasty and fiber-free snack.

To summarize, adjusting recipes for ileostomy-friendly cooking entails picking meals that are low in fiber, simple to digest, and gentle on the digestive system. Individuals with an ileostomy may enjoy a diverse and nutritious diet that promotes their general health and well-being by concentrating on soft, well-cooked products and avoiding foods that may cause pain or obstructions.

To preserve health and well-being while living with an ileostomy, it is necessary to carefully analyze food choices. Individuals with an ileostomy must adjust their dietary habits to meet their specific demands, from hydration to fiber incorporation and special events.

In this section, we will look at several elements of nutrition that are special to ileostomy patients.

Beverage Choices For Ileostomy Patients

Hydration is a critical consideration for patients with ileostomy. It is critical to choose fluid-replenishing drinks that do not increase stool production. Water is the clear option for hydration since it has no added sugars or artificial additives.

Coconut water is another wonderful choice since it is high in electrolytes and quickly absorbed by the body. Individuals should exercise caution while drinking caffeinated or carbonated beverages since they might increase output and cause dehydration.

CHAPTER FOUR
Special Occasion Meals For Ileostomy

Navigating special events may be difficult for ileostomy patients, particularly when dealing with rich, heavy meals. Individuals who plan ahead of time and make wise decisions might enjoy these occasions without feeling uncomfortable.

Lean meats, such as grilled chicken or fish, along with well-cooked vegetables, may create a delicious supper without taxing the digestive system. Additionally, avoiding clear of hot or oily meals might help minimize discomfort and stomach difficulties.

International Cuisine: Ileostomy-Friendly Dining

Exploring foreign cuisine may be an interesting culinary journey for ileostomy patients, but it is important to choose the right meals. Many worldwide cuisines provide tasty alternatives that cater to the nutritional demands of people with ileostomy. Japanese food, for instance, contains sushi and sashimi, which are usually low in fiber and mild on the digestive system. Similarly, Mediterranean cuisine like grilled kebabs and Greek salads uses fresh ingredients that are easier to stomach.

Incorporating Fiber Into The Ileostomy Diet

While fiber is necessary for digestive health, ileostomy patients should exercise caution while consuming it. High-fiber diets may increase stool production, which can cause obstructions or discomfort to the stoma.

Choosing soluble fiber sources like oats, bananas, and cooked veggies may deliver fiber advantages without creating digestive pain. Furthermore, gradually introducing fiber into the diet and monitoring its effects allows people to find a healthy balance for themselves.

Maintaining Weight With Ileostomy Meals

Maintaining a healthy weight is vital for general health, but it may be difficult for ileostomy patients, particularly if they have variations in appetite or nutritional absorption.

Nutrient-dense foods, such as lean proteins, whole grains, and healthy fats, can help you achieve your weight management goals. Additionally, regular weight monitoring and dietary intake adjustments in consultation with healthcare professionals are critical for long-term health.

Increasing Energy Levels Via Nutrition

Fatigue is a frequent complaint among ileostomy patients, sometimes caused by dietary deficits or dehydration. Including energy-boosting items in your diet may assist overcome exhaustion and improve vitality.

Iron-rich foods, such as lean meats, beans, and fortified cereals, help to produce red blood cells and deliver oxygen, thus reducing weariness. Additionally, ingesting complex carbs, such as whole grains and fruits, gives consistent energy release throughout the day.

Hydration Tips For Ileostomy Patients

Proper hydration is essential for ileostomy patients to maintain good health and avoid issues like dehydration. In addition to drinking water throughout the day, integrating hydrating items into meals will help maintain hydration levels.

Fruits having a high water content, such as watermelon, oranges, and cucumbers, contain both fluids and vital nutrients. Additionally, limiting excessive alcohol intake and monitoring urine output might help people correctly assess their hydration state.

Finally, managing nutrition as an ileostomy patient entails carefully selecting beverages, arranging meals for special occasions, and adjusting to different culinary tastes, including foreign food. Incorporating fiber, regulating weight, and raising energy levels via diet are vital parts of preserving health and well-being. By following hydration advice and making smart eating selections, persons with an ileostomy may enjoy a gratifying and healthy diet that fits their particular requirements.

Living with an ileostomy comes with its own set of nutritional concerns. Individuals with an ileostomy must approach their diet with great deliberation and preparation, whether coping with food intolerances, avoiding malnutrition, locating acceptable treats, cooking on a tight schedule, meal planning on a budget, or navigating social settings. This article examines several elements of food management with an ileostomy and provides practical advice for overcoming these problems.

CHAPTER FIVE
Dealing With Food Intolerances And Allergies

To minimize pain and possible consequences, people with ileostomies must manage their dietary intolerances and allergies. Certain meals may cause digestive problems or increase ileostomy-related symptoms.

It is critical to identify and avoid trigger foods by trial and error. Keeping a food journal may help monitor which foods cause issues, allowing for greater control over dietary choices. Consulting with a healthcare expert or nutritionist who specializes in ostomy care may also help you navigate dietary intolerances and allergies.

Preventing Malnutrition With An Ileostomy

Maintaining sufficient diet is critical for general health and well-being, particularly for those who have an ileostomy. The procedure may affect nutritional absorption, thus it is important to eat nutrient-rich meals.

Including a mix of fruits, vegetables, lean meats, whole grains, and healthy fats in your diet will help you acquire enough nutrients. Furthermore, taking supplements as prescribed by healthcare specialists may help address nutritional shortages and avoid malnutrition.

Healthy Desserts For Ileostomy Patients

Individuals with an ileostomy may still enjoy sweets, although with some changes. Desserts that are low in fiber and readily digested might help you avoid discomfort or digestive problems.

Smoothies, gelatin, pudding, and fruit sorbet are a few examples.

Experimenting with different ingredients and recipes may also result in tasty sweets acceptable for persons with an ileostomy.

Cooking For An Ileostomy Under A Time Crunch

Finding time to make meals in today's fast-paced world may be difficult, particularly for those who have an ileostomy and must watch their nutrition. Planning and bulk cooking may be effective time-saving tactics in the kitchen.

Meals may be prepared ahead of time and frozen for later use, ensuring that nutritional alternatives are always accessible, even when time is short. Furthermore, using kitchen equipment like slow cookers or pressure cookers may speed up the cooking process, making it simpler to prepare nutritious meals on short notice.

Meal Plan For Ileostomy Patients On A Budget

Individuals with an ileostomy may eat healthily on a budget if they plan their meals and buy wisely. Prioritizing economical but nutritious meals like beans, lentils, rice, frozen veggies, and seasonal fruit will help you stay on budget while still achieving your nutritional requirements. Planning meals around sale products, shopping in bulk, and making use of store loyalty programs or coupons may all help you save money. Alternative protein sources, like as eggs or tofu, may also be less expensive choices for those with ileostomies.

Socializing And Dining Out With An Ileostomy

Maintaining a social life and eating out may be difficult for people with an ileostomy, but with enough planning and communication, it is perfectly feasible. Before going out to eat, do some research on places that cater to those who have dietary restrictions or specific requirements.

When engaging with restaurant personnel, discussing dietary needs clearly and respectfully may help guarantee a pleasant eating experience. Bringing ostomy supplies and medicines, if necessary, might provide you peace of mind when away from home.

Furthermore, concentrating on socializing rather than just eating might help move the attention away from dietary restrictions.

Conclusion

Living with an ileostomy requires careful consideration of food choices as well as ways of dealing with potential problems.

Individuals with an ileostomy may maintain a satisfying and balanced diet by controlling food intolerances and allergies, avoiding malnutrition, eating nutritious sweets, cooking effectively, meal planning on a budget, and navigating social settings.

Seeking advice from healthcare specialists and engaging with support networks may give essential resources and help manage nutritional demands efficiently.

Individuals with ileostomies may have a varied and fulfilling diet that benefits their general health and well-being with careful preparation and a good attitude.

www.ingramcontent.com/pod-product-compliance
Lightning Source LLC
Chambersburg PA
CBHW070739260726
48660CB00007B/2906